Can I tell you about having a Stroke?

Can I tell you about...?

The "Can I tell you about...?" series offers simple introductions to a range of limiting conditions and other issues that affect our lives. Friendly characters invite readers to learn about their experiences, the challenges they face, and how they would like to be helped and supported. These books serve as excellent starting points for family and classroom discussions.

Other subjects covered in the "Can I tell you about...?" series

ADHD

Adoption

Anxiety

Asperger Syndrome

Asthma

Autism

Cerebral Palsy

Dementia

Diabetes (Type 1)

Dyslexia

Dyspraxia

Eating Disorders

Epilepsy

ME/Chronic Fatigue Syndrome

OCD

Parkinson's Disease

Selective Mutism

Stammering/Stuttering

Tourette Syndrome

Can I tell you about having a Stroke?

A guide for friends, family and professionals

LISA TAYLOR AND SWEE HONG CHIA
Illustrated by Katie Stanton

Jessica Kingsley *Publishers*
London and Philadelphia

First published in 2014
by Jessica Kingsley Publishers
73 Collier Street
London N1 9BE, UK
and
400 Market Street, Suite 400
Philadelphia, PA 19106, USA

www.jkp.com

Library of Congress Cataloging in Publication Data
A CIP catalog record for this book is available from the Library of Congress

British Library Cataloguing in Publication Data
A CIP catalogue record for this book is available from the British Library

ISBN 978 1 84905 495 9
EISBN 978 0 85700 913 5

Printed and bound by Bell & Bain Ltd, Glasgow

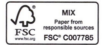

Contents

Acknowledgements

Thank you to our families for their support for us writing this book. Also thank you to our team of proofreaders: Ed, Elizabeth, Nicky, Emma, Sharon, Barnaby and Isabella!

Thank you to Lucy for the editorial support and to Katie for the wonderful illustrations.

Introduction

This book has been written for children and families who are experiencing the effects of a stroke on a loved one. It is written through the eyes of Grandad Fred who has recently had a stroke. It covers what a stroke is and the effects that the stroke has had on Grandad Fred. The effects of a stroke can include problems with physical, cognitive, perceptual, psychological and social issues.

This book is also useful as an educational tool for children and families as to the common early signs and management of individuals who have had a stroke.

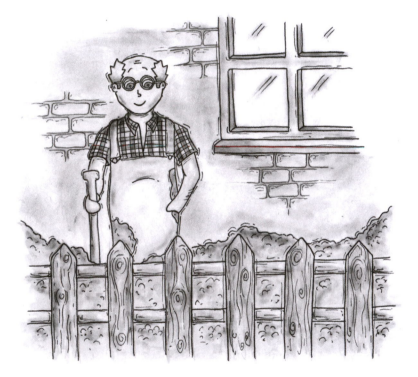

"Hello. My name is Fred, but my grandchildren call me Grandad Fred!"

"I am 63 years old and used to keep myself busy in my garden. I used to watch my favourite football team Norwich City and enjoy ballroom dancing with my wife, Joan. I am going to tell you our story about my stroke.

A few weeks ago I was busy in my garden digging my potatoes. I suddenly had a tingling feeling down my arm. To start with I thought I had done too much digging. But then my leg began to feel weak too. I shouted out to my wife Joan but my mouth felt funny and my words did not come out very clearly. I then began to think that something was wrong with me."

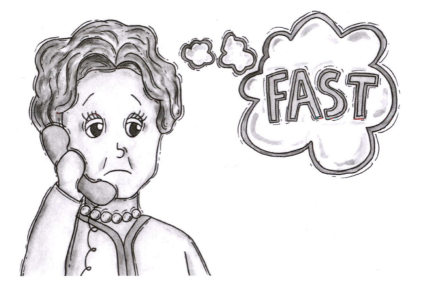

"Joan dialled 999 and we waited for the ambulance to take me to the hospital."

"Joan came out to the garden with a cup of tea. When Joan looked at me and looked at my arm and leg she thought that I was having a stroke. She had seen something on television about how you can tell someone is having a stroke by thinking about FAST:

F – face – has a person's face fallen on one side?

A – arm – can the person raise both arms and keep them there?

S – speech – is the person's speech slurred?

T – time to call 999 if a person is showing any of these signs."

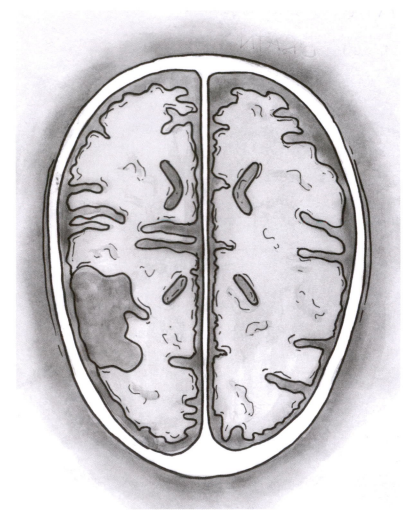

"A stroke happens in your brain."

"The ambulance took me to the Accident and Emergency (A&E) department at the hospital. The doctors wanted to take a picture of my brain (a computerised tomography – CT scan) to see if I was having a stroke.

Your brain normally sends lots of messages to the rest of your body to tell it what to do. Blood flows round your brain through lots and lots of little tubes (vessels). They said that a stroke is when one of the tubes splits and bleeds (haemorrhage) or a big bubble of blood blocks one of the tubes (clot). On the picture of my brain the doctors said that they could see that there was a blockage in one of the tubes in my brain – which meant that I was having a stroke."

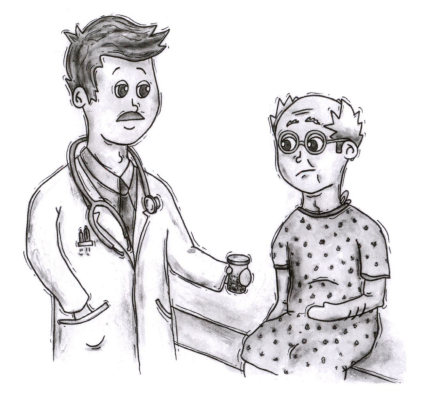

"There was some medicine that I needed
to take to help to get rid of the clot."

"The doctors wanted to try to stop any more damage to my brain. The doctors explained that it was important to find out whether my stroke was a bleed or a clot. If it is a bleed you need medicine to stop bleeding. If it is a clot you need medicine to make the blood thinner (anticoagulant) so that clots disappear. The doctors said that it was really important to take these medicines as soon as possible. They said that it was lucky that Joan realised that I was having a stroke so quickly. Apparently the sooner I took the medicine to get rid of the clot the better the chances of me getting better."

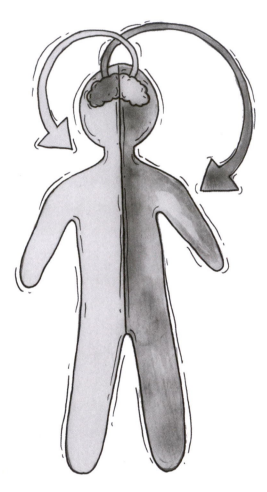

"The brain is split into two halves. Messages from the left side of the brain make the right side of the body work. Messages from the right side of the brain make the left side of the body work."

"The doctors explained that the medicine gets rid of the clot blocking the brain. The blood in our bodies carries oxygen to the brain, which is really important for our bodies to work properly. The clot had stopped the blood going round properly. This meant that part of my brain was damaged where the oxygen had been stopped. We were told that there are areas of the brain that do particular things. The brain can help us move, think, behave and use our senses, such as seeing and hearing, normally. I suppose it is a bit like my football team at Norwich City Football Club – the Canaries at Carrow Road. All of the football team players play in different positions with special skills in those positions – all helping towards the team overall."

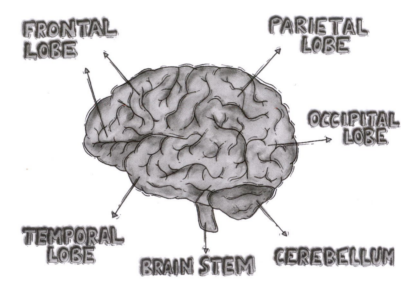

Main areas of the brain

"The main areas of the brain are the frontal lobe, the occipital lobe, the parietal lobe, the temporal lobe and the cerebellum. It depends where you have had your stroke in your brain as to what is affected.

My brain was affected in the left side, which meant that I could not move the right side of my body very well – they called this hemiparesis. Hemiparesis can happen on the right hand side or the left hand side of your body. It would have been called hemiplegia if I could not move one side of my body at all. Because my muscles were a little bit weak my mouth also felt a bit droopy. The damage to my brain also meant that I found it difficult to speak."

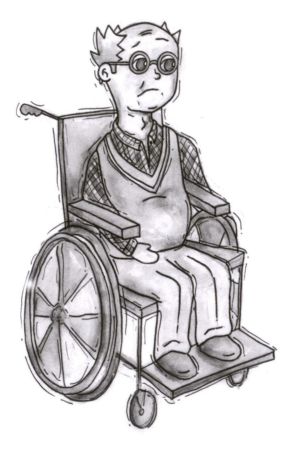

"After the stroke I had to use a wheelchair."

"Anyway, after the visit to the Accident and Emergency department I was moved to a ward within the hospital. I think it was then that I realised that I was not going to be going home very soon! The ward was a special ward for people who had had a stroke. I was put in a bed with my arms and legs in a particular position – which is supposed to help my body. My blood pressure was constantly being checked. I was asked lots and lots of questions. I was really pleased that Joan was there to answer them. This was really tiring for both of us. The staff needed to check where I lived and what my life was like before my stroke."

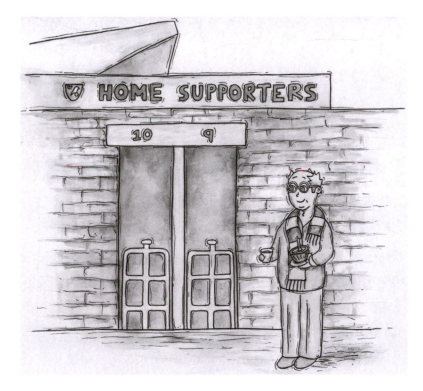

"Before the stroke I loved to go and watch my favourite team."

"Apparently there are certain things that can lead to a stroke, including:

- high blood pressure

- smoking

- poor diet

- lack of exercise.

Thankfully I did not smoke. My ballroom dancing and gardening kept me active. I could have been healthier in my diet – I did like a pie before a football match, and fish and chips on a Friday! I did not know that I had high blood pressure – but I had! It was a real wake-up call having the stroke. I promised myself that I would look after myself from now on. I wish that I had known to reduce my risk factors before my stroke. I realised that recovering from a stroke was not going to be fun."

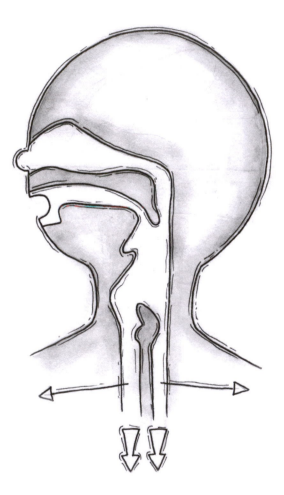

"Swallowing can be hard after a stroke."

"I was feeling really hungry after all of the questions. As I said my muscles were weak – including my mouth. I had to have my swallowing checked to make sure that I did not swallow the food or drink down the wrong pipe. The food or drink should go down the pipe into your tummy. When your muscles are weak, sometimes it can accidentally go down the pipe into your lungs instead (called aspiration). Aspiration makes you cough and can make you ill with a chest infection.

A person called a communication or speech and language therapist came to speak to me and checked that my muscles were working OK. The muscles had to be checked before I was allowed to eat or drink. I was lucky that my muscles were just about strong enough. I had to be really careful that my muscles did not get too tired. If I got tired while eating there was still a risk of my aspirating. I had to have food a little bit at a time, which was really frustrating when I was so hungry and thirsty!"

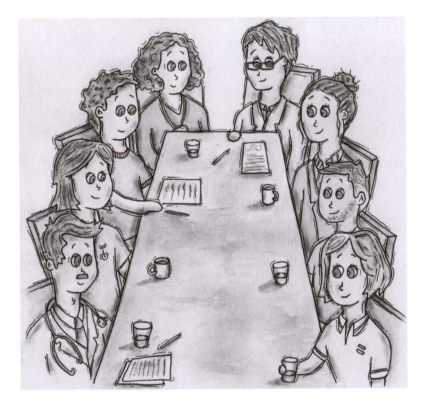

The rehabilitation team

"After a few days on the stroke ward the staff decided that I was ready to move to another ward for some rehabilitation. Rehabilitation is there to help people recover from a stroke. The thing that amazed me about this whole process is the number of people who were involved in looking after me. I will try to explain what the main members of staff do who tried to help me get better. All these people together make a fantastic team."

Doctor

"The doctor had to find out what the matter was with me. Doctors do lots of tests and then decide the medicine that someone needs to try to get better. They work closely with all of the team but particularly the nurses."

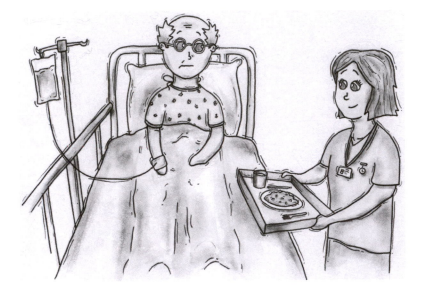

Nurse

Nurses

"The nurses made sure that I took the medicine that the doctors had told me to have (they call this prescribing). They also checked my blood pressure. They also weighed me regularly to make sure that I was not losing weight. They made sure that I was eating and drinking enough. They helped me do my everyday things such as washing and dressing and going to the toilet. I just had to ring my bell and they came to help me. The nurses made sure that they told the rest of the team if there were any medical issues that they needed to be aware of. I think what they developed together for me was called a care plan. A care plan included the medicines that I needed to take, my main problems and what was being done to try to help me with those problems."

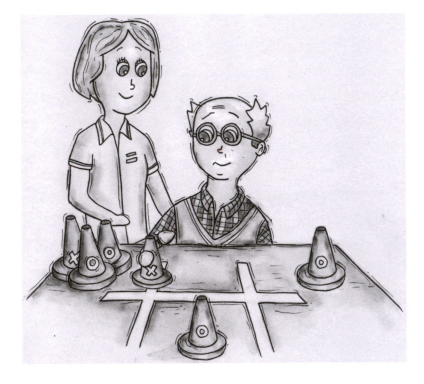

Occupational therapist

Occupational therapist (OT)

"My occupational therapist called herself an OT for short. The OT spent lots of time discussing my house, my family and friends and my hobbies. She also discussed how I was managing to do things for myself before my stroke. I had to show the OT how I could get myself dressed. She wanted to see how I was managing everyday activities now compared to before my stroke. She worked really closely with the physiotherapist and sorted out a wheelchair for me to use while I was not able to walk. She talked through the problems that I was having. We worked together to make some goals for me to achieve during my rehabilitation. The OT used her imagination to come up with some really clever activities that made me work towards the goals we had set without even realising it. The OT also spent time with Joan to see what support Joan could provide when I got home."

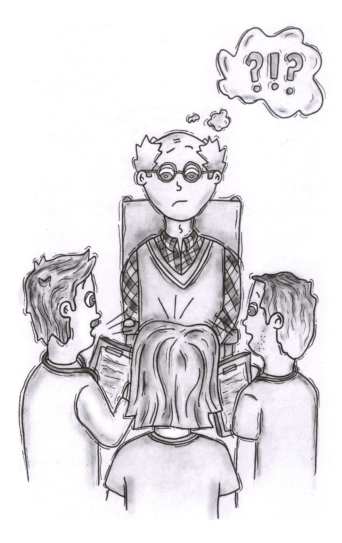

Speech and language therapist

Speech and language therapist (SLT) / Communication therapist

"I already mentioned that I saw the speech and language therapist (SLT)/communication therapist. As well as the swallowing, she wanted to find out what my communication was like before the stroke. The SLT discovered that when people said a lot to me all at once, I had trouble keeping up with what had been said. This problem was worse if a few people were chatting to me at once. The SLT explained the speech and language problems to me and Joan. The ward staff were also told so they could all make sure I understood what was being said to me all of the time. She also gave me exercises to help me remember words more easily. I sometimes found it difficult to find the right words when I was talking with people. (This is called expressive dysphasia.)"

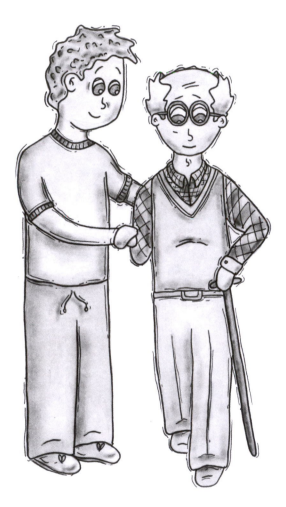

Physiotherapist

Physiotherapist

"The physiotherapist made sure that I was lying properly in bed and sitting properly in my wheelchair. The physiotherapist moved my legs and arms to try to get them to work properly again. I had a really hard exercise programme to try to wake up my muscles again. It was really exhausting and I ended up having a sleep to recover afterwards. Apparently it is normal to feel really tired after a stroke. Joan was also told about what was happening with my muscles. Joan was given some exercises to do with me. This made her feel like she was helping, I think. Just like the OT – we set some goals for me to achieve. Obviously walking by myself was the big one for me. There were lots of little goals on the way to achieving that goal – I had to be really patient!"

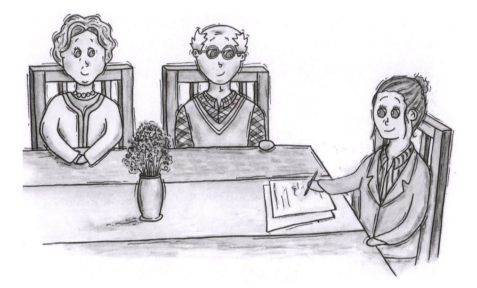

Social worker

Social worker

"The rehabilitation team were not sure if I was going to need help with money matters. The social worker was contacted and she came to talk to me and Joan about our finances. It was really useful to know what funding there is that we may be able to receive. The rehabilitation team also told us they could organise carers to come to my house and help me with washing and dressing if I needed."

Dietician

"I was beginning to lose weight so the team asked the dietician to see me. The dietician gave me some drinks called supplements. The supplements made sure that I was getting enough energy. The dietician also spoke to me about some ideas of what to eat from now on that would be better for my health."

Health care and therapy assistants

"There were a whole group of health care and therapy assistants who were a really important part of the rehabilitation team. These people worked with the therapists and nurses to carry out my rehabilitation programme."

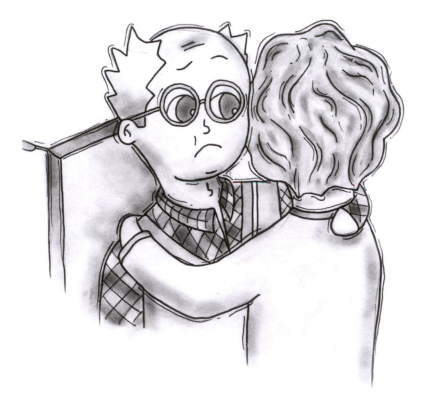

"The weeks of rehabilitation
were really hard emotionally
to cope with sometimes."

"The team were great – and we all worked together to help me work towards my goals. I just wanted to be able to do everything that I did previously. I slowly became aware that life had changed – I think Joan realised it too. We talked about our ballroom dancing and wondered if we would be able to do that again. Although I was able to stand up now with a stick it took so much energy out of me. Also my arm was still not working properly.

The emotional side of a stroke is really difficult to deal with. I found that I would cry – something that I never usually did. The team were really good with supporting me and Joan emotionally. After chatting with the OT about my feelings she gave me a questionnaire to fill in. The questionnaire checked how my feelings were affecting my life – was I feeling very fed up all of the time (depressed) or was I very worried about things all of the time (anxious)? The questionnaire results showed that I was just feeling a bit fed up and missing my old life, which was perfectly normal given the situation."

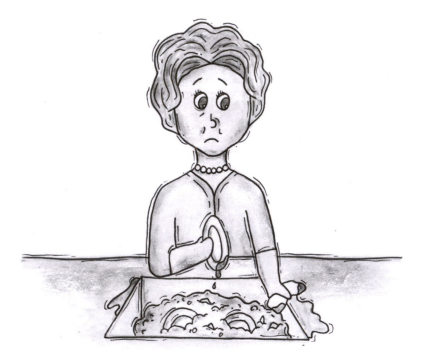

"Joan felt lonely without
Fred being at home."

"I had always been so active before my stroke. I suppose that Joan and I had always had a traditional relationship. I did the DIY, washed the car, did the gardening. Joan did the cleaning, washing and making the meals. I felt bad that I was not going to be able to do my jobs for a while. That did not seem very fair for Joan. The roles we were playing in our relationship were changing and that was difficult to accept.

I was not looking forward to trying to get to the football by myself. Joan hated football and I could not ask her to consider taking me. My season ticket that I have had for 40 years is up some flights of stairs. I would need to be able to walk up steps! Football stadiums are not the easiest places to walk around at the best of times. The crowds bustling past would make me really worried about getting knocked over. Yes, life was going to change big time. I really did want to be able to get to watch my beloved Norwich City if I possibly could."

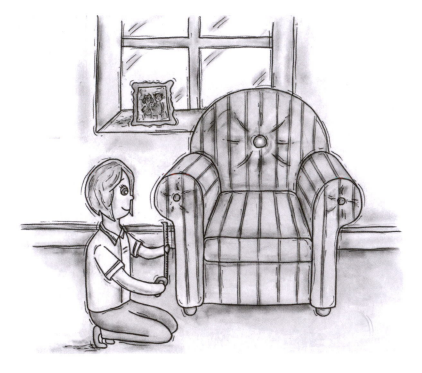

"The OT had already gone out to my house to look at how my wheelchair could get around the house."

"She had a long chat with Joan. They talked about where my favourite chair was, which side of the bed I slept on and whether I prepared meals. Joan and I had a bit of a laugh about the meal preparation – I leave that all to Joan! I think Joan was hoping that I might come out of hospital having learned how to cook a meal! I do like to make Joan a cup of tea first thing in the morning. The OT talked about things that help kettles pour safely and various other pieces of equipment that may help me get back to making Joan her cuppa.

Anyway – I think the OT was able to tell that with a bit of equipment here and there I could return home. I was really relieved as I thought that I was never going to be able to go home. I had really worked hard towards getting home. The people in the hospital are really friendly but I was missing home. I could not wait to sit in my own chair at home. So many people I had met in the hospital had already gone home and I was waiting for it to be my turn."

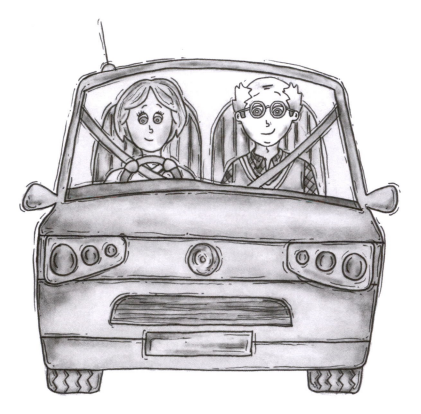

"The team finally decided that I had made sufficient progress to go on a trial visit home with the OT."

"It was really strange sitting in a car again on the way back home. It made me realise how different life is when you are in hospital. There is a completely different routine to being at home. When we arrived home, the OT got various bits of equipment out of the car for me to try. We managed to get into the house – luckily I had a really deep step so the wheelchair was able to get onto it before getting into our house. I think the OT was thinking about putting a ramp there to help Joan get me in and out. Good old Joan was able to push me inside the house just like the OT, so we did not need a ramp. Also I think that they are hoping that I will not be in the wheelchair for too much longer anyway."

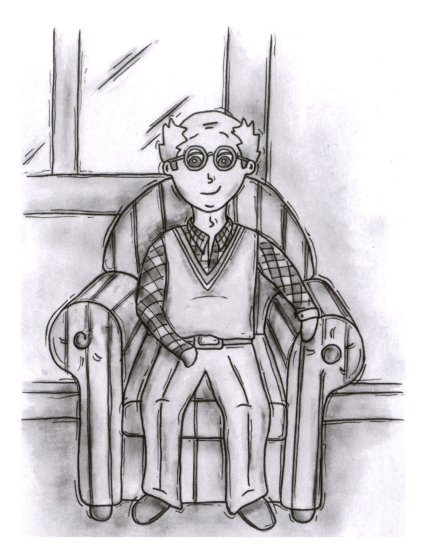

"The greatest feeling was to get
into my armchair! I really felt
great – and realised how much I had
progressed to be able to do that."

"The OT really put me through my paces. I had to get from my wheelchair into my bed (luckily we have a spare room downstairs that I was able to use for sleeping in for the time being). All the physiotherapy sessions practising getting from my wheelchair to a chair really paid off! There were a couple of pieces of equipment that the OT said may be useful. She suggested raising my bed a bit as it was a bit low. There were some really useful bits in the toilet to hold on to when I am getting on and off the toilet. By the end of the visit I was exhausted physically and emotionally. It had been a very successful visit – the OT was happy that I had done enough to be able to return home. That news was really exciting. I was thinking, though, if I am that exhausted from a one-hour visit home – how exhausting is it going to be when I get home properly? I will have to do those activities every day."

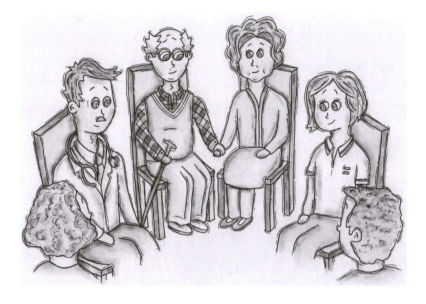

"After the visit home, things really happened quickly – we had a special meeting called a case conference to plan my discharge (going home)."

"The case conference was a meeting
with all of the professionals who had been
involved with me. The meeting discussed my
progress so far and whether I was doing well
enough to return home safely. The decision
was made that I was able to return home but
would need further rehabilitation at home
to get as well as I possibly could. Joan felt
that she was able to help me with some of
the activities that I still needed help with.
The social worker did not need to organise
carers to come in to help after all."

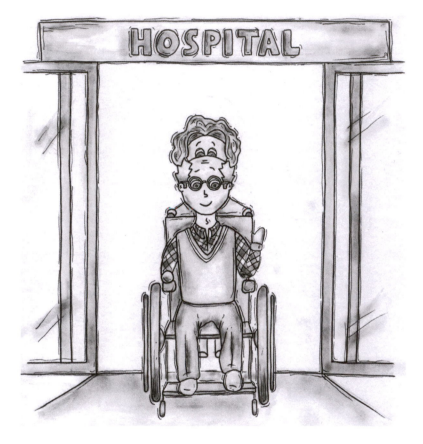

"The team at the hospital were fantastic and really worked together to fix me up enough to get home."

"Before I knew it, I was saying a teary goodbye to the staff. I never usually cry but as I say I think that the stroke has made me a bit more emotional.

The next stage for me was to see if I could continue to get myself even more independent. I wanted to be able to get to do more of the things that I really loved doing. My life was more than just getting dressed, eating and going to the toilet by myself.

Before I left the ward I had been introduced to a community team of therapists. This community team would continue with my rehabilitation when I returned home. I was glad that they had not finished with me yet. I really wanted to be able to walk again by myself and go into my garden! The team said that they would be able to visit me in my own home every week to carry on my rehabilitation."

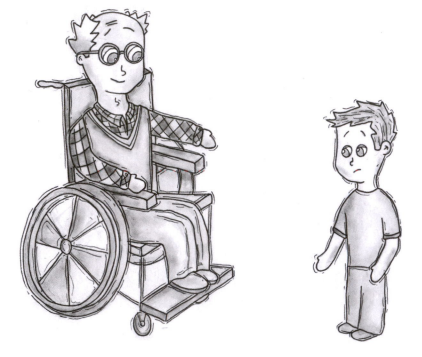

"The grandchildren seem scared to cuddle me in case I break! I keep telling them that I will not break and cuddles help Grandad to feel better."

"I think that we felt that we had a great team helping us when I had my stroke. Poor Joan had to go home to an empty house every night. I thought I had it bad being left in the hospital but at least I had people around me 24 hours a day. Joan was like a rock – the other halves really do hold things together. Joan's life has changed too; she is having to do a lot more to help me than she did before. Joan is getting tired herself visiting every day. Actually the ward staff did say for her to have a day off visiting every now and then. If Joan got tired and ill that would make life very difficult.

I can imagine it can get frustrating for family and friends. Recovery can be very slow and life changes for everybody – not just the person who has had a stroke. My grandchildren used to love gardening with me, and they have not been able to do that."

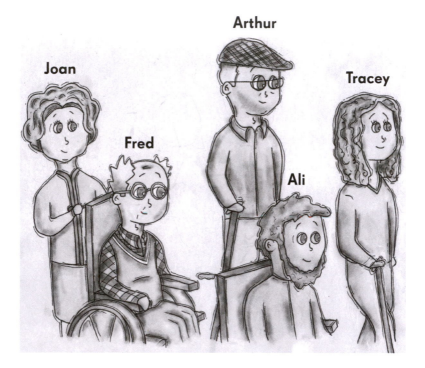

"The physiotherapist suggested a support group that she knew about. The support group met in the community hall every week to provide support to those who had been affected by a stroke."

"We were thrilled that we could go and be able to talk to people who had been through the same experience as us. The support group believes in life after stroke and supports individuals who have had a stroke to make the best recovery they can. The group's activities involve talks from people who are experts on strokes and can offer advice. It was great to share our experiences with others who had had a stroke too.

I met lots of people in the support group, some of them with different problems from me and I have introduced some of them below."

Arthur

"I learned a lot from Arthur. Arthur had a stroke a couple of months before me. Arthur's stroke was in a different area of his brain so he had different problems from me. We just clicked – he was a Norwich City supporter too. Arthur had problems with his memory (a cognitive problem) and also did not notice things on his left-hand side (a perceptual problem). He could pretty much walk by himself and use his hands with just a little weakness. Arthur used to push me round in my wheelchair. The problem was that he kept pushing me into things because he did not notice things on his left-hand side! His eyesight was fine – it was when his brain had to interpret and make sense of what his eyes were seeing that he had a problem – that is, a problem in visual perception. When he was getting the biscuits ready on the plate for coffee time he would just put them on half of the plate and not realise. Arthur's dodgy memory meant that he had to keep a diary with him to help him remember what he was doing and when. It made me realise that a stroke affects different people in different ways.

We struck up a really good friendship and we made a goal that we would go to the football together. It took a lot of thinking about though – going to a football match in a wheelchair is not an easy thing to do. We knew that we would not be able to use our normal seats but really wanted to see Norwich City play again. "

Ali

"Ali was another person who I met at the support group. English was not the language that Ali learned when he was a child. It was really important for the professionals involved with Ali to ensure that he understood what was being said to him. An interpreter was appointed to help with the communication. Ali had got some speech and language problems from his stroke, which resulted in difficulty in understanding what was being said to him (receptive dysphasia). Ali was another person whose stroke had affected him in a completely different way. We learned a lot from Ali and his wife – particularly how different cultures and religions deal with illness in different ways."

Tracey

"Tracey was only 35 years old when she had her stroke. Tracey had problems with the left side of her body. She was able to walk with a stick but her arm was still not moving properly. Tracey has two young children, six years of age and three years old. Tracey's husband (Paul) worked offshore on the gas rigs. This meant that he usually worked away for two weeks and then had two weeks at home. Tracey could not look after her younger child by herself as her arm still did not work properly. Paul had to stop work to help Tracey with the childcare and housework. They did get help from a carer for an hour a day. With Paul not working, the main worry for Tracey was financial. Before her stroke Tracey always did everything with the children. Now things had changed and this change was really difficult to deal with. Luckily there were other groups for younger people who have had a stroke. Tracey also said that her social worker had been great, organising benefits and so forth to help."

"I had my stroke six months ago and I am still making progress. I am now able to walk around our house and garden with a stick. I have been able to go back to driving. I went to the regional driving assessment centre to make sure that I was able to do everything that I needed in order to drive safely. Arthur was not allowed to go back to driving because of his perceptual problems, so I drive him to the football match. We changed our season ticket seats so that we can sit together and we don't have to manage any steps to get to our seats. We have had a stairlift put into our house so I am able to sleep upstairs now – the community OT helped us to organise that. We have still not been able to get back to ballroom dancing. I think we might have to change the type of dancing that we do. We have made new friends through my stroke. We spend time with our new friends, which is really important to us. Life is different after my stroke. We have learned to accept that this is our life now. We need to make the most of what I am able to do and enjoy life as it is now."

Glossary of terms

Cognition – thoughts, understanding and reasoning about the world

Dysphasia – a problem with the understanding or expression of language

Hemiparesis – a weakness on one side of the body

Hemiplegia – a loss of movement on one side of the body

Perception – the interpretation of the information received from the senses

Stroke – a clot or bleed in the brain resulting in an interruption in the blood flow, causing damage

How family and friends can help

- When someone has problems with their speech and language:

  - Remember that, just because they have difficulty understanding, they have not become less intelligent.

  - Treat them as adults!

  - Don't rush the conversation.

  - Write down key words.

  - Try gestures, drawings and pictures.

  - Use short sentences and use them in context.

  - Don't pretend to understand.

  - Be supportive.

  - Make sure the room is quiet.

  - Face each other.

  - Make sure that only one person speaks at a time.

- It is very tiring after a stroke so please allow rest for individuals who have had a stroke.

- Things will take longer to do after a stroke – please allow the person time to do and practise things.

- Recovery will take time and the individual, their family and their friends will need a lot of support in the changes to their lives that are a result of the stroke.

- Individuals can sometimes be more emotional after a stroke and may get more frustrated, angry or tearful than they usually would.

- Please give the professionals as much information as possible about the individual's life before the stroke, as they are able to tailor rehabilitation to the individual.

- Giving measurements and clear information about the home situation will help to plan the discharge from hospital.

- Be realistic about the support you will be able to provide long term, as this will help in the production of appropriate plans.

Professional organisations

Dieticians
The Association of UK Dieticians (BDA)
5th Floor
Charles House
148/9 Great Charles Street Queensway
Birmingham
B3 3HT
United Kingdom
Phone: 0121 200 8080
Email: info@bda.uk.com
Website: www.bda.uk.com/about/about_bda/contact

American Dietetic Association (ADA)
ADA Location Headquarters
120 South Riverside Plaza
Suite 2000
Chicago
IL 60606
Phone: (800) 877 1600
Website: www.diet.com/store/facts/american-dietetic-association

Medicine
British Medical Association (BMA)
BMA House
Tavistock Square
London
WC1H 9JP
Phone: 020 7387 4499
Website: http://bma.org.uk

Royal College of Physicians - National Clinical Guidelines for Stroke
11 St Andrews Place
Regent's Park
London
NW1 4LE
Phone: 020 3075 1318
Email: stroke@rcplondon.ac.uk
Website: https://www.rcplondon.ac.uk/resources/stroke-guidelines

American Medical Association (AMA)
AMA Plaza
330 N. Wabash Avenue
Chicago
IL 60611-5885
Phone: (800) 621 8335
Website: www.ama-assn.org/ama/home.page?&linkid=iw_component-1

Nursing
Royal College of Nursing (RCN)
Copse Walk
Cardiff Gate Business Park
Cardiff
CF23 8XG
Phone: 0345 772 6100
Website: www.rcn.org.uk

American Nurses Association (ANA)
8515 Georgia Avenue
Suite 400
Silver Spring
MD 20910-3492
Phone: (800) 274 4ANA (4262)
Website: http://nursingworld.org

Occupational Therapy

**British Association of Occupational Therapists
and College of Occupational Therapists**
106–114 Borough High Street
London
SEQ1 1LB
Phone: 020 7357 6480
Website: www.cot.co.uk

**The American Occupational Therapy
Association, Inc. (AOTA)**
4720 Montgomery Lane
Suite 200
Bethesda
MD 20814-3449
Phone: 1-800-377-8555
Website: www.aota.org

Physiotherapy

Chartered Society of Physiotherapy (CSP)
14 Bedford Row
London
WC1R 4ED
Phone: 020 7306 6666
Website: www.csp.org.uk

American Physical Therapy Association (APTA)
1111 North Fairfax Street
Alexandria
VA 22314-1488
Phone: (800) 999 2782
Website: www.apta.org

Social Work
The British Association of Social Workers (BASW)
16 Kent Street
Birmingham
B5 6RD
Phone: 0121 622 3911
Website: www.basw.co.uk/england

National Association of Social Workers (NASW)
750 First Street
NE Suite 700
Washington, DC 20002-421
Phone: (202) 408 8600
Website: www.socialworkers.org

Speech and language therapy
Royal College of Speech & Language Therapists (RCSLT)
2 White Hart Yard
London
SE1 1NX
Phone: 020 7378 3012
Email : info@rcslt.org
Website: www.rcslt.org

American Speech-Language-Hearing Association (ASHA)
2200 Research Boulevard
Rockville
MD 20850-3289
Phone: (800) 638 8255
Website: www.asha.org

Voluntary organisations and information

Stroke Association
240 City Road
London
EC1V 2PR
Phone: 020 7566 0300
Email: info@stroke.org.uk
Website: www.stroke.org.uk

American Stroke Association
7272 Greenville Avenue
Dallas
TX 75231
Phone: (1 888) 478 7653
Website: www.strokeassociation.org/STROKEORG

Blank for your notes